You Are Getting a Lung Transplant:

AN EXAMPLE GUIDE

Katheryn Skalet

First Edition

NEWMAN SPRINGS PUBLISHING
320 Broad Street
Red Bank, NJ 07701

First originally published by Newman
Springs Publishing 2025

ISBN 979-8-89308-915-8 (Paperback)
ISBN 979-8-89308-916-5 (Digital)

Printed in the United States of America

I dedicate this to my mom, Jeff Skalet, Paige Crooks, and Abbey P.

Prequel

I have had a chronic lung disease since I was born. I frequently had pneumonia as a baby, as a young child, in my teen years, and in my adulthood. My chronic illness and side illnesses like colds, etc. ultimately led to my diagnosis of bronchiectasis.

A lung transplant is not an easy solution, but it is often the only option for those with chronic lung diseases. The road to qualifying for the transplant list is long and challenging, requiring significant lifestyle changes and medical evaluations.

I had to undergo several medical examinations to determine the extent of my illness and how well my body would respond to the transplant surgery. It was a rigorous process of physical, mental, and medical evaluation, but I knew it was necessary to live a healthy and fulfilling life.

To be eligible for the transplant list, I had to commit to making significant lifestyle changes. This included giving up my social drinking habit, which was challenging, but I knew it was necessary for my long-term health. I also had to undergo several medical procedures, including a colonoscopy and a dental checkup, to ensure that I was in good overall health and that there were no factors that could interfere with the transplant surgery's success.

The evaluation process also involved several blood tests, walking tests, and respiratory rehabilitation to ensure that my body was as strong as possible for the upcoming surgery. I had to undergo dialectical behavior therapy classes to help me manage my stress and anxiety, which was an essential part of the process, as the doctors wanted to ensure that I was mentally prepared for the surgery and the recovery process that would follow.

Overall, the journey toward a lung transplant was challenging, both physically and mentally. It required a lot of dedication and hard work, but I knew the transplant was worth it. When I finally passed all the evaluations and met all the criteria, I was accepted onto the transplant list. It was a significant milestone in my journey, and I knew the next step would be even more challenging.

A lung transplant is not a decision to be taken lightly, but for those who need it, it can be a life-saving procedure. If you are considering a lung transplant or have been recommended for one, know that the journey toward qualification is challenging but worth it. It requires dedication, hard work, and a commitment to making significant lifestyle changes, but in the end, it can give you a chance at a healthier and more fulfilling life.

The journey toward a lung transplant requires dedication, hard work, and a commitment to achieving the best version of yourself. For me, this meant undergoing a rigorous process of physical, mental, and medical evaluation by the doctors to determine if I was a suitable candidate for the transplant surgery.

As someone with a chronic lung disease, I knew that the road ahead was going to be challenging, but I was determined to do whatever it took to qualify for the transplant list. This involved undergoing several medical examinations to determine the extent of my illness, as well as my body's ability to respond to the transplant surgery.

I knew that I had to be mentally prepared for the surgery and the recovery process that would follow, which was why I underwent dialectical behavior therapy classes to help me manage my stress and anxiety. This was an essential part of the process, as I had to be mentally strong to overcome the challenges that lay ahead.

One of the most significant challenges I faced was giving up my social drinking habit. The doctors caught me several times, which was embarrassing, but it was also a wake-up call to make significant lifestyle changes. I knew that giving up drinking was necessary if I wanted to qualify for the transplant list, and I was willing to do whatever it took to achieve my goal.

In addition to the lifestyle changes, I also had to undergo several medical procedures, including a colonoscopy and a dental checkup. The doctors wanted to ensure that my body was in good overall health and that there were no factors that could interfere with the transplant surgery's success. I also had to undergo iron infusions to address my anemia and low iron levels, which was a challenge, but I knew it was necessary to improve my overall health.

The journey towards a lung transplant was not easy, but I knew that it was worth it in the end. When I finally met all the criteria and was accepted onto the transplant list, it was a significant milestone in my journey. I knew that the next step would be even more challenging, but I was ready to face it head-on. With hard work, dedication, and a commitment to improving my health and well-being, I was one step closer to achieving my goal of a healthy life. I was diagnosed with bronchiectasis when I was six years old. My lungs collapsed several times before my transplant; they filled with fluid, and my oxygen level was at seventy-two percent, which is dangerous. By the time I received my double lung transplant at the age of twenty-nine, my lungs were so badly scarred that the tissue adhered to my ribs. Too much info? Well, this book is full of information.

Chapter 1

Getting the News

You have probably been waiting a long time to hear the phrase, "You need a lung transplant."

Qualifying for and anticipating this surgery is more involved than Dorothy's journey on the *Yellow Brick Road*. It is more like a triathlon:

1. The doctor announces the news to you.

2. The doctors will examine your body to determine what it needs and what must be achieved for the surgery to be successful.
3. Exercise is a big one; they may tell you your weight is not acceptable, as they want you to be the healthiest version of yourself for this complicated surgery.
4. Physical therapy is for strengthening your muscles and your existing lungs.
5. Dialectical behavior therapy classes help manage stress and anxiety.
6. They will test you for alcohol and drugs; failing these tests could mean elimination from the list. (I will talk more about this later.)
7. I am getting on the list!
8. They will call you, and then…*surgery time*!

Chapter 2

Doctor Announces the Surgery Is Approved

I had the jitters when I received the news that I qualified for the surgery. They tell you the average lifespan of your new lungs, and it freaks you out because of how delicate the transplant seems. At first, it was just a goal to qualify for the transplant list, but then it became apparent that this healthy lifestyle would be my new passage to life. The doctors came to examine me and informed me that it was a requirement to avoid alcohol and edibles for my chronic nerve pain from small nerve neuropathy. They explained that I might not feel comfortable with my body after my surgery (I will get to that later.) I felt elated—I was on cloud nine, gaining the knowledge of what I had to do to qualify for this surgery. At the same time, I was dedicated to the process, even though it was going to be challenging.

Chapter 3

My Journey Part 1 Qualify to Get on the Transplant List

I had to exercise, exercise, and exercise. The exercise goal was the easiest part. The doctor's team sent me to respiratory rehab. Respiratory rehab is a gym membership with a trainer, which was helpful. Thirty minutes a day of walking because the doctors want your body to be as strong as possible. I aced that part. My problem as a young adult was social drinking, and they caught me several times, which was embarrassing. Part of the process is repeating blood tests. Alcohol can be detected in your system for two weeks. It took me three to six months to commit to that goal of no drinking and realizing living the *party life* is less important than your new lungs.

Once I passed dialectical behavior therapy, which helped control my anxiety and aided in not drinking, I could be placed on the list after I accomplished working out for a long period (which I never thought I could do). I had a colonoscopy and a dental checkup (they do not want teeth falling into your new lungs, ok? I thought it was kind of weird at first too). I had to take walking tests and blood tests. I also had to receive iron infusions because I was anemic and low on iron. Do you know how weird it is to see pure black liquid in an IV tube going into your arm? It's weird! But there are stranger things, I suppose.

When you are campaigning yourself for that surgery, it can feel like you are on a hamster wheel of discomfort. I constantly struggled to breathe, and now I am asked to do a million and one things to be the best version of myself. The doctors will not accept anything less. But the transplant was worth it; at the end of the day, all the hard work finally paid off!

Chapter 4

Accepted on the List!

I received a call a week after being on the lung transplant list. I was getting an iron infusion when I answered the call. The people over the phone said, "Your lungs are here! Go home, pack a bag, and return."

I waited about eight hours upon my return to the hospital for my surgery, as they had to test and confirm the donor's lungs were in good condition. I sat anxiously; no medications were allowed until I went back into the operating room. Finally, I received word that everything was approved, and the transplant surgeons were preparing the surgery room. My husband and mom gave me hugs and kisses, and I was wheeled back for surgery.

My first surgery lasted nine hours. I was in a medically induced coma because my chest cavity was too swollen. My rib cage was exposed, with bandaging wrapped tightly around me. They were unable to close me up due to the swelling. They waited four days until they could stitch me up properly, which also required staples. After I was finally out of the coma and sewn back together, the not-so-fun part began, including hallucinations. I was strapped to the bed so I could not tug or pull on anything. I had drainage tubes coming out of either side of my ribs, as well as a tube coming out of my urine tract and my backside. You don't want me to go much deeper into that part. I had a breathing tube placed to help my lungs keep moving, which was my breathing mechanism. The tube was removed after a couple of days to see if I could breathe on my own, but I wasn't strong enough yet so it was placed back in. The next option was to perform a tracheostomy in my throat so they could use the respirator to help me ease into breathing on my own (my husband told me later that he was terrified about it because of the risks and scarring, but it sped up my recovery so he was glad we did it). Afterward, my mouth felt like cotton—parched. I could not get relief, as I had no pleasure in eating an edible or getting a real sip of water.

The care team had to roll me back and forth to bathe me on a tarp in bed. I had to stand up and sit down for exercise to strengthen my muscles for a few days. I did not have the strength to do any more than that. I had to write on a whiteboard while my hands were tied to a bed, which was stiff and awkward. Eventually, they released my hands so I could sleep properly and write well on the whiteboard. Using the whiteboard was the only way to communicate, as the trach prevented me from speaking unless a voice box was attached. The pain worsened as they decreased the pain medications level by level. I remember being up for tweny-four hours straight (I didn't sleep at night), waiting for Jeff to come back to save me and tell the nurses that I was in pain; I couldn't speak on my own. I thought a nurse had left me in an elevator. Hallucinations haunted me, but it is all part of the lung transplant recovery.

My other hallucinations were rays coming at me from a computer and hurting me. I am pretty sure I saw a famous actor as my nurse. I watched *Beauty and the Beast* and thought it was all in watercolor. I thought my *sister* was someone else who looked exactly like her, and I wrote on the whiteboard to tell her she was my sister's twin. It was my sister! I thought my husband was his brother, which was weird, and that he was hiding in a corner. Those are all the hallucinations I can recall. I do not have hallucinations now; however, with all of the medications I am on, I still experience confusion. The hallucinations pass; do not worry. Since I can get through these odd times, you can too! It may seem scary, but only because it is terrifying.

Chapter 5

Moving out of the ICU to the Transplant Floor

The move to the transplant floor was so gratifying! I could start using the restroom again with assistance. I had a feeding tube placed inside me until the doctors were confident that I could swallow food without choking. My first meal of choice was Chipotle. It was a steak burrito, and it was delicious! *Mmmm.* I can still taste the sour cream. Of course, that could be from the Chipotle burrito I just had…

I did more sitting in a chair as exercise; who knew that would be so strenuous? I walked around the floor with an IV pole and a walker, in pain because they want you to feel the pain so you do not exceed your limits. You, the doctors, and the nurses know you're in pain, but they must know why. Once I gained enough strength on the transplant floor, I rang the celebratory bell three times: one for the donor, one for the whole *sha-bang*, and one for yourself. I was so proud of myself for getting myself to this point.

Chapter 6

The Physical Therapy Floor

The physical rehab floor is for strengthening your body before you go home. After my transplant, there were many games and exercises to improve my body. I would say the most painful part was getting the feeding tube removed and the rib and back pain. I still have mid-back and lower-back pain from the surgery. You will still experience this pain mildly over time. I see a pain doctor and get my nerves zapped so I can't feel the pain in my lower back. Also, removing the trach was weird; it felt strange to have a gap healing in my throat. Upon going home, I could do tasks without assistance, such as eating, drinking, and moving about. I was asked to do laps continuously around the hospital floor. I felt like a lousy athlete going through this whole experience. Finally, after a few days, I was strong enough to climb the stair apparatus in the gym. They had a prototype car I had to practice getting in and out of to strengthen my leg and chest muscles. I did a lot of hand-strengthening exercises as well. My energy level remained strong, so I kept pressing forward, increasing my endurance and muscle strength.

My family often visited, except for my dad, who only visited once. I was happy he came at all, as he was not there for me on the medical side of things. My mother, my husband, my sister, and my cousin were my caregivers. My dad was on the phone and there for me in that way. I love my dad; his can-do attitude made him stop drinking at sixty; he started his own business and moved from Massachusetts to Texas and finally to Colorado, where he made his home. He hated the hospital, so I never blamed him for not participating in my health care. By this point in my life, I was numb to his absence in my transplant journey. Parents should come to support their daughter in the most significant moment of her life—literally life or death. I am not trying to scare you away from this challenging health decision. However, you have a right to know; your transplant team will tell you the risks at the beginning of your journey. Anyway, enough about my father; he had flaws, and nobody is perfect, but he was a good man. I am writing about him not to be disrespectful but to relate to all the other patients whose family members do not participate in their health journey. I know it is a huge letdown, but they are good people with their fears, and at times, they are incapable of helping you deal with all of the complications surrounding chronic illness.

After being released from the physical rehab floor, the next step was to go home! Upon going home, I would be cared for by a village. I still felt alone and sad because I was still like a patient in my home, but I pressed on, knowing a stronger me was on the way.

Chapter 7

Going Home

When I arrived home, my mom practically lived with us for a while and helped with laundry, food, medications, and cleaning! She was my *Wonder Woman*, and my husband was my *Spider-Man*... I'm a female *Deadpool*, healing from the brink of death and writing this book.

Chapter 8

Pain Management

I was discharged to home with my PICC line and a feeding tube was still in place. Being on bed rest was difficult, as I was getting cabin fever. I have small nerve neuropathy, and I was eventually allowed to eat edibles to ease the pain. The edibles helped with the pain in my back, rib cage, and generally all over.

It was complicated for me to shower, and when I could shower, my feeding tube and PICC line had to be hidden and covered. Taking at least twenty-five medications daily is mind-blowing to keep track of on a piece of paper they send you home with. Your family and friends have to adjust to the new glamorous you, as you have many *war wounds* to be proud of as a result of the transplant.

Chapter 9

Neverland Finish Line

Then the doctors had me rejoin physical rehab. That part was fun, but I felt like the youngest person in the hospital gym. I still kept pressing on. I still use cannabis to help with my nerve pain. People may assume I am a healthy person, but they don't see the pain, suffering, diagnosis, waiting for a diagnosis, surviving the disease itself, the transplant, and your near-death experiences relating to the diseases and trial and error of different medicines. It is a lot. Do it, go through it, ring that bell on the other end, and be proud of the life you live. YOLO, you know? Then write a book.

Chapter 10

Making the Difficult Decision

Write a table listing the pros and cons, and consider the decision. Death is inevitable at some point. That is where I made the decision. It was either death by disease or death by trying to get the transplant. I chose to go for it. If one were to think about it and choose differently, that would be perfectly okay. I am not trying to push you into doing it, but it's a chance to live longer. Think about it: if you give the surgery a chance, there is more life to live.

Tools to survive:

- You or a family member should bring music and movies. Unfortunately, you won't be able to cuddle with a stuffed animal due to risk of infection. Plus, all the drainage tubes kind of prevent that from happening anyway.
- If your hospital doesn't have a whiteboard, please bring one because you'll lose your voice. Communication is necessary, and that's the best way I know.
- Meditating and deep breathing will help. You can bring a positive focus object like your stuffed animal, which you can watch from afar.

This surgery is for those who believe they can handle all of the above, but some do not even get past respiratory rehab and its workouts.

If you ask me if I would do it again…I probably would, but I wouldn't want to be selfish and take away somebody else's chance to live longer.

I dedicate this book to my mom and my husband, Jeff, who kept me going during this challenging time. My sister made me dinner, and my cousin visited me to make dinner. I had a village, and that's what it takes.

I hope you choose whatever makes you happy and fulfilled in life.

—Love,
Katie Skalet

Anxiety Guide

DBT methods for anxiety. This is DEARMAN:

1. Describe: Describe what you need to understand their feelings and words without judgment.
2. Express: Use *I* statements to express your feelings so you're not pointing fingers.
3. Assert: Assert yourself calmly to ask for what you want without the other person's judgment or interruption.
4. Reinforce: Reinforce how you feel about the person and treasure them.

The goal is to explain what you wish to do calmly and politely.

5. Mindful: Stay mindful of the present situation to stay on track and calm
6. Appear: Appear confident, sit up, stand tall, and look them directly in the eye.
7. Negotiating: Negotiate a compromise that benefits both parties.

Wise Mind:

Emotional mind vs. Reasonable mind

- Emotional Mind: When your emotions take over rational thinking.
- Rational Mind: Uses only logic, so keep your feelings intact for life skills like flight or fight, for example.

Get yourself in a helpful place by meditating: "This is called a wise mind."

How to Get to a Wise Mind:

1. Pay attention to your breath; you can even think *wise* as you inhale and *mind* as you exhale
2. Ask wise mind questions while you practice breathing
3. The goal is to get to a neutral state for wise and logical thinking.

Mindfulness:

1. Observe and describe.
2. Participate.
3. Just observe sights, sounds, tastes, and what you hear around you.
4. Describe the reactions or symptoms of the paper stress (e.g., chest heaviness)
5. Participate in what you're doing and focus on the task at hand instead of worrying about *what-ifs*.

Wise Mind:

1. Non-judgmental experience of the setting and what's happening; you don't have to agree. Just do not be judgmental and put emotions aside.
2. One mindful practice is focusing on the main subject and letting go of all the distractions around you.
3. Effectively: Be effective towards the goal; avoid focusing on being right or wrong. Think of the solution instead.

TIP:

1. Tip the Temperature: Use cold water or ice to trick your body into adjusting its temperature.
2. Intense Exercise: Engage in activities like jumping jacks or any exercise that makes you sweat and helps you forget.

3. Paced Breathing: Breathe from your belly, not your chest. Go slowly, taking one breath every ten to twelve seconds.

F. Focus on fairness and only facts
A. Apologize
S. Stick to values
T. Truthful

There are more DBT skills on the web! I hope at least these five help you.

PS, Your journey is only your business. What other people see does not even scratch the surface. While healing after a transplant, be patient with yourself; keeping yourself healthy will be a lifelong job.

About the Author

Katheryn Skalet has had bronchiectasis which eventually led to a double lung transplant. She wrote her first book in 2024, *Welcome to the Hospital*, in 2024 for children in hospitals, and then *Pongos World: and His Family* in the same year. Now, she brings you into her lung transplant journey. Enjoy!

www.ingramcontent.com/pod-product-compliance
Lightning Source LLC
LaVergne TN
LVHW101618210926
848480LV00009B/812
9798893089158